Defeat fibroid And Be free

My True Life Story

ONLY THE SICK KNOWS THE IMPORTANCE OF WELLNESS

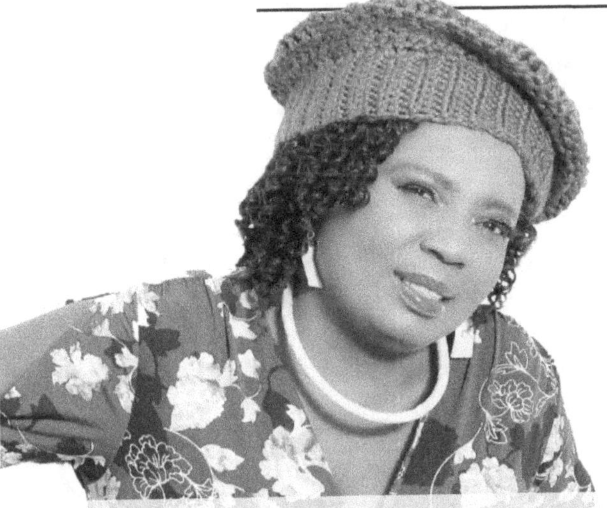

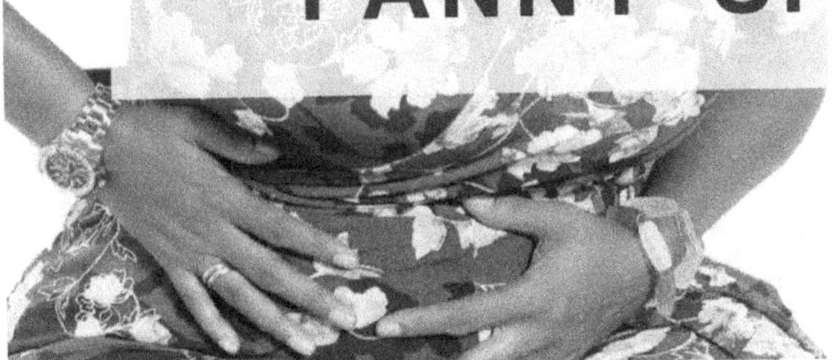

FANNY S. PALMER

My True Life Story

A Patient's Guide for Treating and Managing Fibroids.
An Informative Handbook for Every Woman.

I AM A FIBROID FIGHTER
AND SURVIVOR

I AM AN ADVOCATE FOR THE HOLISTIC APPROACH
TO THE TREATMENT AND MANAGEMENT OF FIBROIDS

Let's Say **No** To
FIBROIDS!

FANNY S. PALMER

DEDICATION

This book is dedicated to Jesus Christ, my Lord and personal Saviour, for saving me from death and His divine healing upon my life. Jesus, You are my Hero.

Jesus, the God of many chances, I thank You for everything. Thank You, Lord, for giving me the opportunity to share my story with the world.

"Bless the Lord, O my soul, and forget not all His benefits." Psalm 103:2

This book is also dedicated to women who are suffering from fibroids.

Also, I dedicate this book to my beloved parents, Mr. Oscar Samuel and Mrs. Cordelia Albertine Palmer, both of blessed memory.

ACKNOWLEDGEMENT

I acknowledge God for redeeming me from my predicaments. I also thank and acknowledge my husband and my family members both at home and abroad. Words cannot express how grateful I am to Dr. Pastor & Mrs. Mensa Otabil, Rev. Kofi Asiedu and the entire International Central Gospel Church (ICGC) Ghana and around the globe. I also want to acknowledge and thank my spiritual fathers in the Lord, His Grace the Bishop & Mrs. Awuradeasem Kofi Darko, Bishop & Mrs. Nat Nketia Mensah and Pastor & Mrs. Albert Mensah in Accra, Ghana. I acknowledge and appreciate Rev. & Rev. Mrs. Jeremiah C. Swarray Snr. of Kingdom Empowerment Ministry and Rev. Hon. & Rev. Mrs. Abraham Sesay Jones of Family Chapel Ministries, Freetown, Sierra Leone. You all stood by me during my predicaments and encouraged me to write this book. I also want to thank and acknowledge Apostle Dr. Mawuli Mawuko,

Rev. Daniel Dankwah, and Madam Eugenia Elikem Abena Kumage, all in Accra-Ghana, for proofreading the manuscript of this book. I want to acknowledge Dr. David Jalloh in Freetown, Sierra Leone, who stood above all odds and treated me when others gave up on me, and also for proofreading the manuscript of this book. Also, I acknowledge and thank my very dearest coach and friend, senior coach Ariel, the Wellness Coach of Ariel's Haven in Accra, Ghana.

An acknowledgement to Prophet & Mrs. Joseph Kofi Nyatefenya Zowonu and members of International Grace Calvary Ministry and also Pastor & Mrs. George Bassaw in Accra, Ghana.

Finally, I acknowledge my boss Mrs. Mariatu Bangura, Chief Officer at the Ministry of Social Welfare in Sierra Leone. Thanks to all my friends, fans, and the Body of Christ in Sierra Leone and Ghana. I also appreciate my dearest daughter and sons in the Lord, Pastor Hawa Bangura, Pastor Yusif S. Caulker, Pastor Guastavus Jones King and Minister John Idriss. You all have played an essential role in my life's journey. I profoundly appreciate and value your love and support beyond description. May God bless you all!

Disclaimer

I admit that I am neither a medical doctor nor a medical practitioner, and this book is not a medical book. Therefore, the views expressed herein are the culmination of my personal research on the treatment and management of fibroids, coupled with my personal experiences with fibroids.

CONTENTS

Dedication   v
Acknowledgement   vii
Preface   xiii

Chapter 1
My Journey With Fibroids   1

Chapter 2
The Woman Internal Anatomy And
Fibroid Growth   13

Chapter 3
Menstrual Period And Fibroids Development   19

Chapter 4
What Are Fibroids? Types And Causes
Of Fibroids   25

Chapter 5
Signs And Symptoms Of Fibroids   33

Chapter 6
How I Almost Died Of Fibroids   37

Chapter 7
How To Defeat Fibroids And Be Free   51

Chapter 8
Self-Care & Wellness Practices To Manage
Fibroids   59

Chapter 9

30 Prayer Points For Feminine Wellness
Against Fibroids   69

Chapter 10

31 Days Wellness Affirmation Scriptures To
Comfort Fibroids Patients   73

PREFACE

How can I defeat fibroids and start living a happy life again? This is one of the most frequently asked questions by women suffering from symptomatic fibroids. The pages in this book contain the secrets of how I have lived with symptomatic fibroids for several years. They also contain the methodologies that I discovered through books, articles, and YouTube videos that are related to the treatment and management of fibroids.

This book has been presented in a readable format so that women who suffer from fibroids can learn about other alternative methods of managing fibroids and also learn how to defeat and be free from them.

I hope you discover an answer to your fibroid condition in this book. Additionally, you will understand the meaning, signs and symptoms of fibroids, which are key in the fight against fibroids,

The quest for finding a solution to the fibroid condition became obvious in my late thirties, so I started reading books and articles on the topic. I also watched YouTube videos that are related to fibroids to empower myself on how I could win the fight against fibroids. On the other hand, some patients with fibroids shared with me similar painful stories they had experienced with fibroids, which inspired me to write this book.

As the Bible says in Hosea 4:6, "My people are destroyed for lack of knowledge." This book, among other things, is to raise awareness of fibroids at the community, national and international levels; also, to empower and raise support for girls and women suffering from fibroids. It is high time for women to stop being ashamed or silent about their fibroid conditions.

Despite fibroid conditions being common among women, women with fibroids are still overlooked by most authorities at the national and international levels. They forget the fact that many women are losing their precious lives to this horrible condition and that something must be done to save our lives; because women suffering from fibroids' lives matter too.

This book also serves as a guide for sensitization about fibroids and a tool to raise awareness for institutional support from governments, agencies, departments, Offices of the First Ladies, the World Health Organization (WHO), non-governmental organizations (NGOs), and religious and traditional authorities to advance research on fibroids; also, to provide adequate funding, medical services and to develop policies that will help save women suffering from symptomatic fibroids.

This book is also obligated to stir up open discussions about the inclusion of the fibroid condition as a reproductive healthcare concern; because women's fertility and wombs are in jeopardy, which is a threat to procreation; likewise, to raise awareness about male and female fertility because just as some women are facing challenges in conceiving, some men are also facing challenges in impregnating women.

Women play a vital role in productivity and reproduction, and as such, our health should be prioritized from all angles. Women with symptomatic fibroids suffer in silence because most people are not aware of the negative health implications they inflict on girls and women, and as a result, most of them do not empathize with us or give us much emotional support as compared to women suffering from breast cancer.

Since July is observed annually as fibroid awareness month, therefore, I call on all individuals, groups, organizations and institutions to throw their support for girls and women suffering from fibroids by wearing white dresses a day or a week in July to show their support for women and girls suffering from fibroids.

I encourage everyone, but most especially men to be very supportive of their sisters, mothers, nieces, daughters, wives, co-workers, female friends and neighbours who are suffering from symptomatic fibroids.

Likewise, I wrote this book to break the silence and stigma associated with fibroids and menstrual periods in our communities, and most especially in our religious settings, as **fibroid and menstrual periods are two sides of the same coin**. Many women with symptomatic fibroids are suffering in silence because of these cultural and religious beliefs associated with menstruation. Leviticus 15:19-25-28.

Fibroid is a life-threatening condition which sometimes renders some women infertile. Some women also have ectopic pregnancies which occasionally lead to maternal deaths. Symptomatic fibroids are causing some women to unintentionally absent themselves from work, some children to be motherless, some husbands to be widowers, and marriages to be broken beyond repair. It as well breaks down women emotionally, psychologically, socially and financially.

Many women are losing their uterus (womb) to fibroids, and some have mask-up smiles but are silently suffering from this medical condition. Fibroid does not literally kill women, but its symptoms may lead them to their death, especially in the case of unattended prolonged heavy bleeding. Some women die or suffer from complications during or after fibroid surgeries (myomectomy/ hysterectomy).

Some women with bigger fibroids can experience leakage of uncontrollable urine. This condition is called urinary incontinence, and it negates the woman's quality of life. Some women will even develop lower abdomen bulges which portray them as pregnant women, and all these are embarrassing situations for women and girls.

Women are expected to bear children within their reproductive age, but the evil spirit (fibroid) finds this period the best time to attack and most times, prevents women from conceiving. O! What a double pain some women had to go through. That is why we should not be quick to judge, condemn or make a mockery of women without children; for you may not have the slightest idea of what they are going through. Whenever you see a woman desperately looking for the fruits of the womb, pity her; do not be like "Peninnah", but always remember that the God of "Hannah" is still alive and can still bless women with fibroids if it pleases Him. 1 Samuel 1:27

Bible tells us about the woman with an issue of blood. Most of us are familiar with that scripture but have no idea of what she went through; only women suffering from symptomatic fibroid can fully relate to this passage in the Bible. This book is a fibroid awareness book which aims at empowering women suffering from fibroids to rise and speak about their condition because fibroid conditions sometimes affect women's mental health.

I wrote this book to share my story in order to preclude many more women from losing their lives to fibroids, and also help those already suffering from it because fibroid condition is a secret killer.

"My people *(women)* are destroyed for lack of knowledge" Hosea 4:6. To me, a fibroid is like an evil spirit that thrives on the ignorance of women, and most women are held captive because of lack of knowledge about the condition. Fibroid is from the pit of hell and must be treated holistically, medically, naturally and spiritually through prayers.

Personally, I deem fibroid as an evil spirit because it manifests itself just as Jesus said about evil spirits, "When an evil spirit is cast out, it goes and comes again." When a woman is diagnosed with symptomatic fibroid, it becomes another new chapter of pain and discomfort.

The Bible says; the devil comes only to steal, kill and destroy (John 10:10). And that is how fibroid operates in a woman's body. Whenever it attacks a woman, her quality of life changes, and if not managed well, it kills the woman or destroys her future. That is why I say "Fibroid is an evil spirit".

I liken fibroid to an evil spirit because when a woman is diagnosed with symptomatic fibroids and decides to go for an operation (myomectomy), even if she survives the surgery, there is a possibility that within two to three years, this evil spirit will come back, meaning the fibroid will grow again with its symptoms. As Matthew 12:43-45 says, "The evil spirit will return to its original place".

If you are passionate about women's health, this book is for you. If you are a political leader, religious leader, opinion or traditional leader, this book is for you.

If you are a father, mother, uncle, brother, sister, aunt, nephew, niece, cousin, wife or husband, this book is for you. If you are a woman of childbearing age, this book is for you. If you are suffering from fibroids or know someone with the condition, this book is for you. Share this book with others and encourage them to read it. The story in this book is non-fiction with flashbacks.

CHAPTER 1

MY JOURNEY WITH FIBROIDS

One beautiful day in my mid-twenties, I was informed by my doctor that I have developed uterine fibroids. My gynaecologist, by then, was Dr. James Samba, popularly called Dr. Samba. This happened at the 34 Military Hospital in Freetown, Sierra Leone. I found out about the fibroid condition through prenatal examinations. It was the most shocking and disturbing day of my life, as I had never heard of the word "fibroid". After the medical examination, he sent me to go and do a pregnancy test and pelvic ultrasound.

When the results came out, he announced, **"Congratulations, you are pregnant and going to be a mother. However, I have worrisome news for you; you have been diagnosed with**

tiny multiple uterine fibroids, but no cause for alarm, during your delivery, we shall conduct Caesarian and myomectomy sessions, so go home and let's watch and wait". I was confused and tried to process the information at that moment because I could not grasp what he was saying.

After a few months of pregnancy, I had a miscarriage. According to my doctor, the fibroids had put pressure on the baby resulting in the miscarriage. I was so heartbroken. After some months, I gathered some courage and determination to try for another baby. I then discussed it with my doctor, and he recommended that the only way for easier conception was to do a fibroid surgery.

Since I wanted to have a baby at that time and there were no other options given to me for the treatment of the fibroids, I began to pray about it. As a young lady, I began to ask myself, what will I do? What if the surgery was not successful? What would happen to me after the myomectomy? How did I get these fibroids? So many questions ran through my mind at that moment and I needed some answers. I then decided to discuss the fibroid condition with some female family members and friends, but they could only share with me very little information, which was not helping me in my fight against the fibroid all because of the secrecy surrounding our menstrual periods and the lack of knowledge about the fibroids condition.

After several months of battling the fibroids, I finally decided to see Dr. Samba and informed him about my readiness for the surgery/ myomectomy.

I had the surgery done on me and by God's grace, it was successful. I was hopeful that I would conceive again within the following year.

Indeed, God being faithful, I was blessed again with the fruit of the womb, but unfortunately, I had another miscarriage because the fibroids had returned and affected the pregnancy. After a few months of that painful experience, my doctor encouraged me to go for another surgery /myomectomy since I wanted to try for a baby again.

As usual, I went for the second surgery and it was successful. Dr James Samba conducted the first two surgeries on me at the 34 Military Hospital, Freetown, Sierra Leone.

After the second surgery, I was desperately looking for other options from numerous doctors, but they all suggested that I should have another fibroid surgery. However, after several months of praying and searching for alternative treatments, I finally decided to continue with my doctor who had already suggested another myomectomy. Hmm! I had to go for the third surgery at his private hospital which was then located near Jesus Is Lord Church at Tower Hill, Freetown, Sierra Leone.

I became pregnant again after the third successful surgery, but alas, I lost it again to fibroids. I became very heartbroken and was exhausted financially, psychologically, physically and emotionally.

I was a living ghost. I felt wearied every day, and the quality of my life began to deteriorate as I battled with fibroids. I would bleed as if I was going to die at any moment and I was constantly anaemic.

According to my doctors, the normal blood level (haemoglobin) of a female should be between 11.6 to 15 grams per deciliter (g/dl) but in my case, most times, my blood level was between 7 to 8 grams/dl, and the most painful thing was that, as I was taking blood tonic to replenish the lost ones, I will be losing the blood again through prolonged bleeding. It was like pouring water into a leaking bucket. Sometimes, because of the heavy bleeding, I did not feel like stepping out of my house, and the safest place for me was inside my room. If you are a woman and you have been suffering from prolonged bleeding, you can relate to this very well. On some days, I even carried with me an extra dress, pants and pads for any emergency or heavy bleeding, whether in my menstrual period or not. Hmmm! It was not easy for me at all, but by God's grace, I am still on the course to fight against fibroids.

I could vividly remember that fateful day when my colleague at the Ministry of Social Welfare Gender and Children's Affairs, called Hawanatu K. Koroma, informed me about a medical team that was conducting fibroids surgeries without cutting. I was super excited because that was the first time I heard about a different option for treating fibroid rather than cutting my body every time. I gave it some thought for several months and prayed about it also. Within those months, I endured a lot of pain in my body. When the pains and symptoms became unbearable, I gave in to the "No cutting surgery".

I went for the first "No cutting fibroid surgery," making it the fourth surgery in a row, and the surgery was successful. I was confidently sure that this time around the fibroids had been finally uprooted, but after a while, everything changed, I was re-diagnosed with the fibroids.

I then went for another "No cutting fibroid surgery," which was successful as usual, all with the hope of getting a solution to this death trap. I call it a death trap because when a woman is diagnosed with symptomatic fibroid, she is between life and death. She will be trapped, and if no proper treatment is given to her, she might end up losing her womb or life.

Hum! God has really been my Helper all those years of infirmities. The Bible says, "Many are the afflictions of the righteous, but Lord delivers him from them all." Psalm 34:19.

I thought the battle was over after the fifth surgery, but it wasn't. I began to experience the symptoms of fibroid again after some months.

As time passed, my pain and discomfort worsened. The situation got worse day after day, and I felt drained as I was having prolonged and irregular periods accompanied by heavy bleeding. The quality of my life was disrupted from normal to abnormal because of the symptoms of fibroids.

Most times, because of the fear of blood leakage and abdominal pains, I would intentionally call off my participation in some public activities, like family gatherings, weddings, naming ceremonies, parties, church services and work. Also, because of the frequent urination at night, I was having sleepless nights, so, at day times, I used to feel sleepy, which affected my productivity at work.

I remember sometimes in the morning, my younger brother, Oscar Jr. when taking off for work, would call me and ask, "Sister, are you still at home? Why are you not going to work? Why are you sitting at home while your colleagues have gone to work?"

"I'm not feeling well." I would respond.

"But you were looking fine yesterday night, so why all of a sudden this morning you are sick? How come?" he would ask again.

"I just had my period with heavy pains," I would again respond, but he would not understand me. He would just accept it as it was and would say, "Ok, take some medicines and rest."

This was our regular conversation anytime he would see me absenting myself from work. To him, it seemed normal because I am a woman and should be seeing my periods, but little did he know that I was suffering from fibroids, and because of the cultural taboo of secrecy regarding the period, I found it difficult to discuss it with him.

This is how exactly husbands, friends and family members see it, to them, it is normal when their wives, daughters, nieces, mothers, and grandmothers complain about heavy periods and pains.

Whenever you hear a woman complain about heavy periods or menstrual pains, show some concern and encourage her to get medical attention because symptomatic fibroids can be fatal if left untreated.

Here is a great question, "What one thing can you do to save a girl or woman who is suffering from fibroids if you learned about her condition?

Another major effect of fibroids on my life was that there were times I could not wear white or plain bright-coloured dresses. I could carefully select a type of dress to wear when stepping out of the house, but hmmm! White dresses were a no-go area for me.

I would deliberately choose black, brown, or dark mixed-coloured dresses in order to avoid any embarrassment, just in case I happened to leak blood.

Oh my God! I cannot fully give details of the amount of money that I have spent on treatment and medications just to be free from fibroids and yet, I couldn't get any positive results. My journey with fibroids has helped me to fully understand the pain, suffering, and discomfort that the woman with the issue of blood went through. That scripture is my reference point when it comes to my journey with fibroids.

Based on my experience with fibroids, I would like to submit that the woman with the issue of blood in the Bible was suffering from fibroids. Although the Bible did not mention her condition, I deem her a fibroid fighter. You will agree with me if you have experienced fibroids or have knowledge about their signs and symptoms. Matthew. 9:20-22, Mark 5:25-34, Luke 8:43-48.

When a woman develops symptomatic fibroids, stress or grief are some of the great weapons that slowly eliminate her happiness because living with symptomatic fibroids is very stressful.

I used to mask my face with a smile in public, but at home, I was constantly weeping like a baby because of the pain. Most people around me never knew what exactly I was going through except for a few close family members and friends.

I strongly remember one Sunday morning when I woke up with blood clots all over my bed because my period had come unexpectedly.

In fact, on that day, I was supposed to minister in the church as it was a children's day service. Why shouldn't I go to church? It was a special program, and the church was expecting me to be in attendance, so I had to call my younger sister Ranso to help me get ready. She cleaned my room, dried up the floor, and then I put on my mask of pretence and went to church.

Throughout the service, I was still bleeding under my dress while waiting for the time to minister. The most amazing part was that I had been feeling very weak since morning, but the moment the microphone was handed over to me to preach, the Lord renewed my strength, and the pain just disappeared. Hallelujah!

My younger sister, Ranso, was in the congregation, and after the service, she ran to me.

"I had been wondering and saying to myself, was this not my sister who was crying bitterly of pain at home not too long ago? But see her jumping and dancing on the altar as if nothing had happened", she said.

"Sister, I was so afraid of what could have happened to you on the altar if that pain had come again", she continued.

I just smiled because I did not understand it myself, but I knew it was the power of God which helped me out there.

In conclusion, living with symptomatic fibroids is like living in hell. It is not a good place to be. My dear, let's work together to kick fibroids out of our women's lives and put genuine smiles on our faces.

Living with symptomatic fibroids is depressing, embarrassing and incomprehensibly traumatic. It was a painful experience for me because I had to visit several doctors at both government and private hospitals, and sometimes, I bled for a whole year non-stop. I also sometimes pass out (syncope).

You cannot imagine that there was a point in my life when I stopped using normal menstrual pads and started using adult diapers because of the heavy bleeding. To add fuel to the fire, I was later diagnosed with an ovarian cyst. Hum! What a pain we women can harbour and still manage to take care of the family, go to work, attend church services and more. That was how my life was. I was devastated but managed to stand up for others.

I have suffered from symptomatic fibroids for over fifteen years of my life. My journey with fibroids had been a living hell on earth. Having symptomatic fibroids is a life of uncertainty because you never know what is going to happen the next moment.

I used to crave ice blocks, so I became very addicted to ice blocks that I could chew several cups of ice blocks a day. Sometimes, if I decide not to chew ice blocks, I will be very restless throughout the day. Initially, I did not know the reason why I was chewing ice blocks frequently like that, but later on, from my research, I got to understand that it was because of the iron deficiency in my body due to the prolonged heavy bleeding and anemia.

I got married with the desire of raising my own two children in a healthy and godly home like my parents, but my childhood dream was shattered by fibroids as I lost three of my pregnancies to fibroids including my twins.

The issue of fibroid condition is like an open secret, which is unconsciously kept under the carpet while many women are secretly suffering miserably from fibroids.

One thing that baffled me was that, in those days, I hardly found someone to openly talk about my fibroid condition with. It was also difficult to start a discussion around that subject. But thank God for the internet. Today, on YouTube, you can watch many women who are battling with fibroids sharing their stories. To be living with symptomatic fibroids is tough and heartbreaking, and it is just like having a nightmare every night.

CHAPTER 2

THE WOMAN INTERNAL ANATOMY AND FIBROID GROWTH

Several aspects of the woman's internal anatomy are directly connected to her fertility, conception, pregnancy and childbearing. The vagina, uterus, fallopian tubes, ovaries and cervix are the main organs that make up the woman's reproductive system which is the internal female anatomy. The uterus is the major part of the female anatomy that is directly affected by fibroids.

The Bible says: *"Then the Lord God made a woman from the rib He had taken out of the man, and He brought her to the man. The man said, "This is now bone of my bones and flesh of my flesh; she shall*

be called "Woman" for she was taken out of man".
Genesis 2:22-23

From the above scripture, it is evident that the formation of the woman's body is complex and different from that of a man; no wonder the woman is a difficult creature to be completely understood.

Nevertheless, thank God for science which has helped us to have a clue of how the woman's body works. Many people, including women ourselves, sometimes, find it difficult to understand how we really are.

Who is a woman?

A woman is an adult female human. A woman is God's gift to the world and a valuable asset, and when treated with love, care, respect and attention, the world gets the best out of her because we WOMEN ARE SPECIAL. The Bible says: "I praise you because I am fearfully and wonderfully made; marvellous are your works and I know that full well" Psalm 139:14.

"He who finds a wife finds a good thing and obtains favour from the Lord" Proverbs 18:22.

"Behold, you are beautiful, my love, behold, you are beautiful! Your eyes are doves behind your veil. Your hair is like a flock of goats leaping down the slope of Gilead" Song of Solomon 4:1

The above scriptures perfectly describe a woman. God, in His infinite wisdom, thought of the plan to form a woman's body from the ribs of Adam.

THE WOMAN'S UTERUS/ WOMB

The uterus/womb, like a pear-shaped organ, is a hollow muscular organ in the female body. The uterus keeps an egg fertilized and nourished till it is time to give birth. Without the uterus, a woman cannot see her menstrual period. The uterus is of great value for the procreation of mankind.

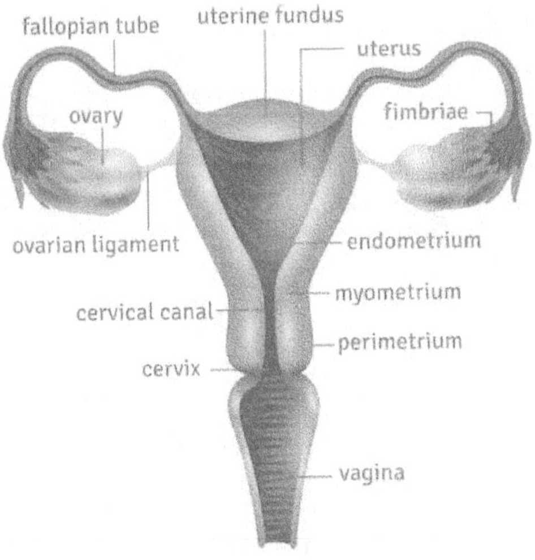

Credit To: Freepik.com/free-vectors

Anytime I see a woman or a girl in their reproductive age, I see a possible victim of fibroid because every woman or girl with a womb is a potential candidate for fibroids. It will surprise many to know that even virgins that are in their reproductive age can also develop fibroids.

THE FEMALE EGG QUALITY BY AGE

Bible says: "My people are destroyed for lack of knowledge" Hosea 4:6.

Research has shown that female fertility is determined by age but with God, all things are possible. A Woman can still conceive at any age if it pleases God, just as He did for these women in the Bible: Sarah, Hannah and Elizabeth.

"And did you know that your cousin Elizabeth conceived a son in her old age" For nothing is impossible with God" Luke 1:36 – 40

Do not be discouraged if you desire to have a child. In fact, you are not too old, like Sarah in the Bible. The table below is to serve as a guide for women who have a history of fibroids in their family to make the right decision regarding childbirth.

WOMEN'S EGG QUALITY BY AGE

AGE   PRENANCY RATE

20-24 years…......................86%

25-29years…..................... 78%

30-34years…..................... 63%

35-39years…..................... 52%

40-44years…..................... 36%

45-49years…...................... 5%

50+…....................…......……0%

Always consult your doctor before jumping to conclusions about your fertility. Couples must partner together when it comes to the issue of fertility because some men may also experience difficulties in getting a woman pregnant. Some possible medical conditions affecting women's fertility are: fibroids, polycystic Ovary Syndrome (PCOS), endometriosis, blocked fallopian tubes, infections, failure to ovulate and more. And for men, they suffer from unhealthy sperm, low sperm count, poor quality sperm, immature sperm and blockage in the tubes of the reproductive system. Also, other health conditions like gonorrhoea, diabetes, infections and more.

So I encourage men to lay aside their egos and cooperate with their female partners and adhere to the doctor's advice for treatment, and also, if possible, look for other possible options for having a baby, like In Vitro Fertilization (IVF), Intrauterine Insemination (IUI), Artificial Insemination (AI) and more. According to doctors, when it comes to fertility issues, the earlier the better for women because of the quality range of the woman's egg by age. So, my dear brothers, uncles, nephews and friends, don't leave fertility issues on the laps of your wives alone. Even if it has been proven scientifically that you are fertile, kindly give her the needed emotional, financial and spiritual support until you both achieve your dream of having a baby by God's grace.

CHAPTER 3

MENSTRUAL PERIOD AND FIBROIDS DEVELOPMENT

"For the life of the flesh is in the blood" Leviticus 17:11. From the above scripture, it is clear that our blood holds our lives.

What is a Menstrual Period? And why do women/girls have them?

A Menstrual Period is a discharge of blood from the uterus. It is the shedding of the lining of the uterus or the endometrium, and it must occur once every month. Whenever pregnancy fails to occur, it leads to a period, that is why women and girls have their periods.

"Menstrual period", "menses", "menstruation", "red rally", "time", "moon", and "red party", are all terms given to the menstrual period, but whatever name you choose to call it, is fine. For common understanding, I will call it 'period or menses' throughout this book.

Some of the symptoms of menstrual periods are; pains, mood swings, dizziness, vomiting, back pain, pelvic pain, headaches, chest pain, muscular cramps, loss of concentration, distress and loss of appetite.

There are a lot of misconceptions and myths surrounding periods. In some countries, it is a taboo for women to openly talk about their periods, not to talk of "men" having discussions about periods. But a lot has changed over the years since the inception of the internet, although some people, especially Africans, still hold on to their cultural and religious beliefs about the discussion of periods.

It is about time we start talking about our periods without restrictions, just as we can talk about our gender, food, football, fashion and others because a period is a natural biological process. Secrecy is greatly associated with menstural periods. Some people think periods are dirty and shameful, forgetting the fact that it is natural for every woman to see her period, and we women should be able to speak about our periods without restrictions.

Even in this 21st century, some educated elites still have little or no understanding about periods and make a mockery of women and girls during their periods, especially when a woman or a girl has unexpected or accidental periods and stains her dress with it. It is very important to understand the situation of women and girls during their menstruation.

More awareness needs to be raised about how to take proper care of women and girls during their periods, especially at our homes, schools, colleges, offices and organizations. In fact, everyone needs to be involved because it is always a difficult time for most women and girls when they are on their periods. I am saying all of this because fibroids and periods are two sides of the same coin, and that is why we need to make every effort to morally and financially support women and girls during their periods.

You may want to ask why women should be supported financially. It will shock some men to know how most women suffering from symptomatic fibroid spend more money on menstrual pads or pampers. Nowadays, some women and girls use menstrual cups to prevent the leakage.

SIX MENSTRUAL PERIOD COLOURS

The colours of the menstrual period blood flow are very important indicators of women's health. The colour indicates whether the period is healthy or not, or if there are pelvic inflammatory diseases, infections and so on. Women should not take the colour of their period for granted. Consult your doctor whenever you see changes in your period.

1. A Bright Red colour period is considered to be healthy and fresh blood flow.

2. A Pink colour period is a sign of anemia, ovulation, low estrogen, unhealthy diet, or weight loss.

3. A Brown colour period is the start or end of a period or early sign of pregnancy.

4. A Black colour period is a sign of a vaginal blockage, old blood, or the start or end of the period.

5. An Orange colour period is a likely implantation or infection.

6. A Grey colour period is a sign of bacterial vaginosis.

NORMAL AND ABNORMAL PERIOD

The woman's body is like a super in-built machine with dynamic functions and parts. The normality and abnormality of women's periods also depend on healthy or unhealthy lifestyles. Thus, negative, toxic or positive environment, food, drinks and medicines. Periods can range from short or long, light or heavy, all depending on the factors that I have named above. Also, periods change as the years go by from age to age, or level to level in every woman's life. Periods can be unstable and fluctuate because of the above factors.

Normal/Regular Period: Usually, the normal period lasts between 3 to 7 days. A period is considered normal when menstrual fluid lost in every cycle is between 5ml to 80ml, and the menstruation is not painful.

Abnormal/Irregular Period: If a woman loses over 80 ml of menstrual fluid (blood) in a month (cycle), it is considered abnormal bleeding. And if the flow comes with cramping clotting and pains, it is a sign that something is wrong in or around the uterus.

Remember that our body speaks to us, so every woman or girl should be observant of the colour of her menstrual period to know whether it is normal or abnormal period.

SOME CAUSES OF HEAVY BLEEDING IN GIRLS AND WOMEN

It is very important to consult your doctor whenever you notice any changes in your period because only a doctor can help you with an accurate answer through a medical diagnosis. Likewise, you must understand that fibroids and endometriosis do have similar signs and symptoms like prolonged or heavy bleeding, pelvic pain, anemia, lower leg and back pain, and difficulties in conceiving a baby. Studies have proved that some women suffering from fibroids may likely have both fibroids and endometriosis at the same time, making diagnosis confusing.

Below are six common causes of heavy bleeding or prolonged bleeding among women:

1. Fibroid
2. Polycystic ovary syndrome(PCOS)
3. Endometriosis
4. Uterine/ Cervical cancer
5. Trauma / Scars in and around the uterus
6. Sexually transmitted infections (STIs)

CHAPTER 4

WHAT ARE FIBROIDS? TYPES AND CAUSES OF FIBROIDS

Fibroids, myomas or leiomyomas are benign or non-cancerous, abnormal growths of the uterus that usually develop during women's childbearing age. Normally, at this age, the estrogen level in women and girls is high.

It can grow in different sizes and locations in or around the womb/ uterus. The size of fibroids can range from lemon seed to watermelon, depending on the location of the fibroids.

I can define fibroid as a female reproductive monster. It is commonly called uterine fibroids, but I will be calling it fibroid(s) in this book for common understanding.

25

Six types of Fibroids

Fibroids are classified according to their locations on the uterine wall:

1. Pedunculated Submucosal Fibroids

2. Submucosal Fibroids

3. Intramural Fibroids

4. Subserosal Fibroids

5. Broad Ligament Fibroids

6. Statunascendi/Cervical Fibroids

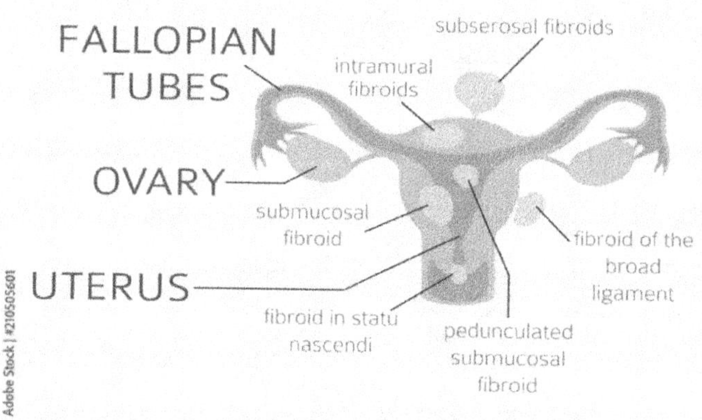

Credit to Adobe stock 210505601

1. Pedunculated Submucosal Fibroids: These types of fibroids are located on a stalk that grows into the uterus and outside the uterine wall.

2. Submucosal Fibroids: Are located beneath the lining of the uterus. It grows inside the uterus and the open space and may develop a stalk in the cavity of the uterine wall. These types are uncommon and develop in the middle muscle layer of the uterus.

3. Intramural Fibroids: Are located in the thick wall of the uterus (myometrium). They grow within the muscles of the uterus wall. These are the most common types of fibroids among women. It can grow big and stretch to the womb.

4. Subserosal Fibroids: These types of fibroids can grow very large, and sometimes, they can have a stalk or root attached to the uterus. They normally grow outside the wall of the uterus. This type is also common among women.

5. Broad Ligament Fibroids: These types of fibroids are double-layer that is attached to the lateral portions of the uterus to the pelvic sidewalls.

6. Statunascendi/Cervical Fibroids: These types of fibroids are located in the cervix, thus, the neck or lower part of the uterus.

Causes of fibroids and Statistics on fibroids

Scientists have not yet found out the exact causes of fibroids. So far, there are no specific causes of fibroids. Its causes are unclear and UNKNOWN, but several factors may lead to fibroids.

However, studies have found that certain women are at greater risk of developing fibroids. The National Institute of Health (NIH) in the United States of America estimated that "80% of all women will develop fibroids at some point in their lives. Since most women do not experience any symptoms, it is possible that the number of women with fibroids is even higher. 20 – 25% of women in their reproductive age have fibroids. By age 50, up to 80% of black women and up to 70% of white women have fibroids. Some studies have revealed that there are about 75% of women that are living with fibroids. I strongly recommend that every woman go and see a doctor as soon as possible for early diagnosis and treatments.

FOUR SIZES OF FIBROIDS

1. Tiny Size Fibroids - very small in size. E.g. lemon seeds.

2. Small Size Fibroids - 1cm to 5cm. E.g. Strawberry to big guava size.

3. Medium Size Fibroids - 6cm to 10cm. E.g. lemon to Apple size.

4. Large Size Fibriods - 11cm and above. E.g. Pear to watermelon size.

RISK FACTORS OF FIBROIDS

1. **Heredity/ Genetic** - If there is a history of fibroids in a woman's family, there is a likelihood that female members from that family may develop fibroids. These women are three times at higher risk of developing fibroids.

2. **Vitamin D Deficiency** - Women with low vitamin D are also most likely to develop fibroids in their lifetime.

3. **Over Weight/ Excessive Body Fat** - Women who are overweight (obese) and inactive are at risk of developing fibroids.

4. **Unhealthy Life Style Without Detoxifications** – Less or no exercise, drinking of alcohol, inadequate sleep, eating lots of macaroni/ spaghetti and indomie/noodles, lots of red meat, eating plenty of carbohydrates without a lot of vegetables and fruits, eating lots of high-fat

(unhealthy) dairy products, may lead to hormonal imbalance.

> Dairy products are products from animals or their milk. Animals like goats, cows and sheep. Examples of some grocery unhealthy dairy products are: clotted/whipped cream, milk, butter, buttermilk, ice cream, yoghurt, cheese, custard, processed meats, and processed foods. Living unhealthy lifestyles by eating these high-fat products and not detoxifying the body can cause inflammation and trigger fibroid to grow or worsen the fibroid signs and symptoms.

5. **Origin/Race:** Many women of African and African-American descent are also likely to have fibroids in their lifetime.

6. **Early Menstruation -** There are possibilities that girls who start their menstruation/periods at an early age between 10 years to 14 years may likely develop fibroids.

7. **Stressful lifestyle:** Most women who are constantly under unhealthy stress have the possibility of developing fibroids. This is because the brain may send signals that throw off the balance of the hormones in the uterus, triggering fibroids to develop.

8. **Pregnancy:** Some women may likely develop fibroids during pregnancy, and they may grow rapidly because the hormone levels will become high, causing the size of fibroids to increase.

CHAPTER 5

SIGNS AND SYMPTOMS OF FIBROIDS

Signs and symptoms of fibroids may differ from patient to patient, depending on the location and size of the fibroids. The two conditions of fibroids are Symptomatic Fibroidsand Asymptomatic Fibroids.

TEN SIGNS AND SYMPTOMS OF FIBROIDS.

1. Heavy bleeding, sometimes with lumps during menstrual periods. This is the most common symptom.

2. Prolonged/abnormal menstrual periods for more than a week or non-stop, making it difficult to track periods.

3. Bleeding in-between menstrual periods.

4. Severe cramping during periods.

5. Frequent urination.

6. Miscarriages and Fertility Problems.

7. Lower back and leg pain.

8. Anemia/dizziness/fatigue/low energy

9. Constipation.

10. Abdominal Distention.

The most confusing thing about fibroids is that some women can have fibroids for years and may not experience any signs or symptoms. In fact, most women may not know that they have fibroids except through a medical pelvic examination by a gynaecologist. Some women may only know about their fibroids condition when they are pregnant through prenatal examination.

When Should a Woman Get Worried About Fibroids?

A woman should get worried about fibroids when she starts having heavy or unpredictable bleeding that affects her day-to-day activities or quality of life, having longer periods than seven days, or bleeding between her periods.

When to Have a Fibroid Surgery?

If a fibroid is not worrying you, do not worry about it, but if you begin to experience severe symptoms and it starts to affect your quality of life or fertility, then you have to discuss it with your doctor about trying other possible options, and if you have tried them but are futile, then you can decide to have surgery.

So, my advice to you is to do your own research and be knowledgeable about other possible options. Also, discuss it with your doctor so that both of you can find the best option rather than just going straight for fibroid surgery because surgery is not the only best option to treat fibroids. From my research, most fibroid experts believe that surgery should be done when the fibroid is between 9-10 centimetres or about 4 inches.

TWELVE FACTS ABOUT FIBROIDS

1. You are not alone. If you are suffering from symptomatic fibroids, know that you are not alone because there are thousands of other women suffering from fibroids.

2. Women between the ages of 30 to 40 years are most likely to have fibroids. However, any age can have fibroids as long as they are in their reproductive age.

3. Myomectomy and hysterectomy are not the only options to treat fibroids.

4. Hormonal imbalance can fuel fibroids. Excess amounts of estrogen in the woman's body can cause fibroids to grow. There should be a balance between the estrogen and progesterone level in the body.

5. Women can still get pregnant with fibroids depending on the size and location of the fibroids.

6. Fibroids are not cancer. They are noncancerous tumours.

7. The exact causes of fibroids are unknown.

8. Fibroids can be managed successfully.

9. Fibroids are diagnosed medically through pelvic scanning/ultrasound.

10. Fibroids cannot be transmitted from person to person.

11. Fibroids are not sexually transmitted diseases.

12. Fibroids are most common in black women than in white women.

CHAPTER 6

HOW I ALMOST DIED OF FIBROIDS

"Yea, though I walk through the valley of the shadow of death I will fear no evil, for the Lord is with me, your rod and your staff will comfort me" Psalm 23:4.

One day in 2015, I heard that some foreign medical doctors were in the country performing all sorts of surgeries including fibroids. The hospital was outside the capital of Freetown, so some days later, I took off to that hospital for the fibroid surgery. The surgery was conducted after a few days, and I was discharged and then returned to Freetown, where I was living by then.

Then one fateful evening as I was sitting outside on our veranda, I felt a liquid running down my legs.

I called my younger sister Ranso to help me out. She held my hands and took me to my room. She then realized that the leaking liquid was not blood. She said, "It is like water flowing," I asked her again to confirm, and she said, "Yes, it looks like water". I laid down for her to check which part of my body the water was coming from.

After she had checked, she said, "Sister, the water is coming from the place where the operation was done".

I then asked her to call Mabel, a neighbourhood nurse. When Nurse Mabel came, she examined me and noticed that the water was flowing down from my abdomen as the operation stitches had gone loose.

Oh my God, another episode had opened in my life! She cleaned me up and applied some first aid and bandaged my abdomen. The nurse, Mabel, advised that I go to the hospital as early as I could the next morning.

Around 1:00 am, the water began flowing again as if someone had opened a floodgate on me. By then, my bedding had become very wet and was giving off a bad odour.

I became very restless and started throwing up throughout that night. My family members in the house could not sleep that night, as they were all worried and started praying for me seriously.

Early the next morning, my younger sister, Ranso, called one of my brothers in the Lord, Pastor Jeremiah Sawray (Sn). In a short time, he was in our house. At that moment, I became so weak and unable to walk on my own again.

My brother infracted traffic rules that day, running at high speed with the emergency lights on. He was issued four tickets (fines) for breaking traffic rules that day. We went from hospital to hospital, and all this happened in 2015 just after the Ebola outbreak in Sierra Leone, so out of fear of the Ebola virus, many doctors and nurses were afraid to see or touch patients, so they were just referring me from hospital to hospital.

By the grace of God, one doctor finally allowed me into his clinic and after examining me, he said my case was above him. So he gave us a referral letter and addressed it to one Dr. Strassar Nicol' at the Princess Christian Maternity Hospital (Cottage hospital). My brother had to drive back from the West end to the East end of Freetown where we were sent to see the said doctor.

Unfortunately, the doctor that I was referred to had retired from the service. If it was not for the Lord who was on my side, I would have died on the way to the hospital.

Fortunately for me, another doctor called Dr. David Jalloh was in the Out Patient's Department. He said, "I do not normally sit in the Out Patient's Department." But God planned it so well that we met him at the Out Patient's Department that day. He quickly came out and asked the nurses to bring me for examination. By then, the fluid was still running down from my abdomen and had soaked the back seat of my brother's car.

After he had examined me, Dr. Jalloh informed my relatives that I had a surgical site infection, so I need to be admitted for proper medication.

I was then admitted to Dominion Ward 2 at the Princess Christian Maternity Hospital (Cottage Hospital), Freetown. My health condition was so serious that it drew the attention of almost all the doctors working at the Cottage hospital. I was at the point of death. But I knew my Redeemer lives. He will neither leave me nor forsake me.

Dr. David Jalloh sent me to do scans on my abdomen. I went for the scans and when the results came, it showed that I had fluid accumulation, a sign of sepsis according to the scan.

I started developing bedsores as a result of the fluid leaking from my infected site. The smell of the fluid became very offensive that I was transferred to a private ward.

I could see scowls on the faces of the people, which was indicating that my condition was getting worse day after day. I became so anaemic that my doctor recommended that I had blood transfusions. I then experienced a negative reaction of swollen face, hands and feet as a result of the blood transfusion. It was not easy for me at all. I know that whiles I was on that sick bed, many people were constantly praying for me, and some had dreadful dreams about me; that I died, that I was in a coffin, that I had been covered with a black bed sheet, that I was buried. Some strangers said they had visions from the Lord asking them to pray for me as I was in a critical condition. Let me use this opportunity to say again, thank you Lord and thanks to all who were praying for me at that time. May God continue to bless you all. Amen!

One day, as I was lying on that sick bed while my sister and sister–in–law had gone out of the ward to buy food, I saw one of my close college mates who was a friend, the late Zainab, who had died long ago, standing at the door of my ward calling me to come to her. I then tried to get up, and when I got up from my bed to go and meet Zainab, I saw my exanimate body lying on the bed, and from nowhere, I felt a strong force pushing me back to my exanimate body on the bed. It was as if I was dreaming, but it was real.

Then on one faithful day after lying on that sick bed for several weeks without any improvement in my health, Dr. Jalloh decided to operate on me to see if he can fix the problem of my infected intestine. He said that, he had a sleepless night that day as the Lord ministered to him to take the risk and to operate on me that very day because I am one of His choicest servants, and my mission on earth has not been accomplished, if not I would die that day.

My faith was neither weak nor strong in those moments, though my body was tired from all the pain. I desired death at some point, but the Lord kept holding my hands.

One day, something shocking happened to me. For the first time in my life, my mind went blank, and I totally forgot about my achievements, status, family and friends. I forgot about everyone and everything. As the Bible says, "for the living know that they will die, but the dead know nothing and they have no

more reward for the memory of them is forgotten."
Ecclesiastes 9:5.

I walked through the valley of the shadow of death, as
the Bible says, "Yea, though I walk through the valley
of the shadow of death, I will fear no evil: for thou
art with me; thy rod and thy staff they comfort me."
Psalm 23:4.

After a few days, Dr. Jalloh prescribed a nasogastric
(NG) tube for me. The prescription was given to my
family members, and they asked my younger sister,
Ranso, to go and buy it at the pharmacy. She went
with all hope to buy it from the nearby pharmacy,
but surprisingly, she could not get it from all of the
pharmacies around, including the hospital pharmacy.
She said, "I roamed about the city for about three
hours asking from one big pharmacy to another but
could not find any. I became tired and wanted to
return to the hospital, but then I started hearing your
voice around me saying 'Save my life, keep on asking"
She said she picked up fresh zeal and started asking
around again, and lo and behold, she saw one small
old pharmacy and said to herself, let try this last one.
As soon as she asked for the nasogastric (NG tube),
the pharmacist went to the shelf and brought one
dusty package, wiped it and showed her the cost.
She added that she was very surprised that the price
of the NG tube was so low; she paid for it and took

Honda (okada) straight to the hospital. She said that the family members in the hospital were all worried about why she had kept long, and she narrated everything to them and they praised God for getting some at last.

My stomach was swollen as if I was eight months pregnant, but immediately the nasogastric (NG tube) was fixed through my nostril into my stomach, a green fluid started coming out of my body through the NG tube, and about two litres came out from my stomach in less than thirty minutes.

By this time, my family, church members, and other well-wishers were saying prayers on my behalf. God directed Dr. Jalloh with fresh ideas about how to handle my case. Nurses revealed that patients with similar conditions had died on the same bed that I was lying on. Other people also dreamt of seeing me in the grave, in a coffin and cage, and there were more of such dreams. I remember when my videographer, Brother David Aruna, told me that he had dreamt of me and that people were covering me with a black bed sheet and telling him that I was dead. He said, he immediately tried to call me on the phone, but could not get me, so he became very worried and went to his church prayer meeting and asked that they should pray for me.

Also, a woman of God who used to stay in low-cost housing in Freetown, came one day to visit me at the hospital through Pastor Jeremiah. Though we were not familiar with each other, she said that while she was on her personal prayer time, she had a revelation about me and the Lord asked her to pray for me.

At one dawn, Dr. Jalloh came and stood by my bed and said, "Today I will take you down", referring to the operation theatre. According to my doctor, my chances of surviving were 50/50. When I was taken to the theatre, I was given anaesthetics through my spine, but when the operation started, I began to feel the pain. Then, the doctor stopped and prayed again, and they gave me the general anaesthetics which caused me to sleep off completely throughout the operation.

According to my sister, Ranso, the surgery lasted for about four hours, and during this time, Pastor Jeremiah and other people were praying for me because I almost died during the operation.

My sister recounted to me that after I was brought out of the operation theatre and then regained consciousness after some hours, I was closely monitored throughout that night by the nurses. When I started recovering gradually, I learned how to walk, talk and write again as the multiple surgeries had affected me so severely; I was fed with tea and water through a 20ml syringe for weeks because I was unable to open my mouth to eat or drink.

A day before I was discharged, I was advised by my doctor not to take my bath because the operation site might open. So for six months, I did not take my bath. My younger sister Ranso used to wipe my body.

Then, I came to appreciate how blessed we are to be able to take our bath as often as we want without any restrictions because some people are in their sick condition and cannot take their bath as they will want to, join me and SHOUT thank You JESUS   !

Within two months in 2015, I had two major surgeries on me, but thank God, I survived it all. I say I AM A SURVIVOR.

Since the operation site was not stitched because of my unstable condition, I was discharged with some bandages wrapped around my waist to prevent the operation site from opening, and blessedly for me, I began to recover faster than expected. When I went for my post-surgery review, I was administered a local anaesthetic on my abdomen. The doctor stitched the operation site, cleaned my wound, put some medicine on me, bandaged the wound and let me go home.. This procedure was conducted at the wards, but not at the operation theatre. It was about four times within two months, and to God be the glory, my doctor completely stitched the operation site neatly and I became free again to take my bath as I wanted to. Alleluiaaaaaaaaaaaaa! Amennnnnnnnnnnnnnnnnnnnn!

Subsequently, because my recovery was faster than expected, my doctors and others were amazed and glorified God for my life. My Doctor, Dr. Jalloh could not hold back his joy and came to our church to testify about the goodness of God in my life, His miraculous healing and the speedy recovery that I had within that short period. He said that the spirit of the Lord came to him one night, telling him that I am His daughter and that he should take the risk to do another surgery on my intestines to save my life. He said that it was like the story of Daniel and King Darius in the book of Daniel 6:18b-19. "And the king could not sleep. At the first light of dawn, the king got up and hurried to the lion's Den."

Dr. Jalloh said, he could not sleep that night, and at first light of dawn, he came to see me at the hospital. "I am glad that I was able to obey God and did the operation on her. I want all of you as a church to know this and remember my words that "Fanny's mission on earth is not just in Sierra Leone; she will cross borders and be a blessing to other nations. She survived for a reason, and you will all see it. I pray that we will all live long enough to see it manifest in Jesus' name."

My doctor told me that, he saw the fibroids but could not remove them because my condition at that time was very unstable. He said, "It is possible for you to conceive a baby because you are very fertile, but you will need regular medical supervision, emotional support and care." He advised me to stay away from stressful lifestyles and situations, as it may affect my healing process and have psychological effects on me too.

I have battled with fibroids for over fifteen years of my life, and it nearly wrecked my life as it was sucking the life out of me gradually.

People gave up on me but God did not. Those who saw me on that sick bed will continue to testify and glorify God for His hand upon my life.

God delivered me, and I want you to keep your faith and believe that with God, all things are possible. He will deliver you no matter your situation. He may come late because He wants to make it big so that His name will be glorified.

By the grace of God, I had a good support system from my family, friends, workmates and other well-wishers. My brother in the Lord, Pastor Jeremiah, supported me financially, morally and spiritually. My siblings, Oscar Jr., Ranso, and my sister-in-law, Augusta, all stood by me and gave me lots of support and words of encouragement, which I needed at that time. I have realized that some people die of sickness because of discouragement and a lack of moral support from family and friends. So I will advise that do not wait for people's funerals before you show how much you care and love them, but rather, give people encouraging words and support when they are sick or alive.

I vividly remember how my sister-in-law, Augusta, used to say to me several times "Mummy do not give up, we need you."

As my health condition worsened, when some of my friends and family members came to visit me in the hospital, some could not recognize me anymore as the sickness had swallowed me up. I remember some stood by my sickbed and asked me for myself. Can you imagine?

They said, "we are looking for Fanny. Where is she? Meanwhile,they were standing beside my bed. My younger sister,Ranso, replied to them, " this is Sister Fanny that you are looking at." Some burst in tears and ran out of the ward in shock.

One day, coincidentally, as my father was walking towards my sickbed, the oxygen concentrator (oxygen machine) that was fixed on me automatically stopped working upon seeing that ugly scene my dad just collapsed. He was rushed out of the ward and was resuscitated.

Oh my God! I vividly recall the day I was in the wheelchair going for the surgery. As the nurses were pushing my wheelchair, I saw my brother, Pastor Jeremiah, he stood by the theatre door. When I saw him, I said in my heart that I would gather strength and hug him as this will be his very last time of seeing me alive.

In the twinkling of an eye, he rushed towards me and shouted, "The devil is a liar, you will not die in Jesus' name". He looked into my eyes and said, "My dearest sister, God is in control. Your mission on earth is not yet completed. Go for your surgery in the name of the Lord. You will come back alive, and we shall all glorify God with you." This is not your last hug, OK.

We are all here praying and waiting for you to come back from that operating theatre alive. " Amennnnnn

CHAPTER 7

HOW TO DEFEAT FIBROIDS AND BE FREE

Scientifically, fibroids can be managed or treated either through conservative surgical or non-surgical approaches. The management and treatment of fibroids varies from patient to patient, depending on the age, location, size and severity of the fibroids. That is why fibroid patients must always consult their doctors for the best medical advice and available options for the treatment of fibroids.

Estrogen and progesterone play important role in the development and growth of fibroids. From my studies, both must be balanced, especially if you are trying to manage fibroids. Also, diet changes can be of great help as well as stress management. Most of the time, symptomatic fibroids normally make life unpleasant for women because it affects the woman's quality of life. The family life, relationships, jobs and productivity of women are greatly affected. So to be free from fibroids and start living a happy life again, it takes a lot of effort and courage.

From my personal experience and knowledge, there is no single way to defeat fibroids and be free from them, that is, they must be treated and managed holistically.

Below are the ten ways to defeat fibroids, be free and start living a happy life again.

Normally, the first three are the most common ways that doctors possibly will prescribe for patients to be free from fibroids and start living happily again. These first four methods of treating and managing fibroids are scientifically proven.

FOUR SCIENTIFICALLY PROVEN METHODS TO TREAT AND DEFEAT FIBROIDS

1. Myomectomy- This is the removal of the fibroids from the womb. This treatment can be very effective, but most times, the "FIBROIDS CAN REGROW."

2. Hysterectomy - This is the removal of the womb, which will permanently stop the fibroids from regrowing. Note that there are different types of hysterectomy.

3. Uterine Fibroid Embolization (UFE) / Uterine Artery Embolization (UAE) - This is the process of blocking the blood supply causing the fibroids to shrink. (NOT TOO COMMON IN AFRICA).

4. Acessa Procedure/Radiofrequency Ablation- This is a new technological treatment for fibroids in which energy is applied through a small needle and destroys the tissue of the fibroid, making the body to reabsorb these dead tissues without any negative effect on the body. Ultrasound and radiological procedures are other methods of treating and managing fibroids. (NOT TOO COMMON IN AFRICA).

TEN NON-SCIENTIFIC PROVEN METHODS TO MANAGE AND DEFEAT FIBROIDS

1. Do nothing about the fibroids. With this first option, doctors normally tell the patient to 'watch and wait'; this is where you will hear the doctor saying, "Your fibroids are tiny or small, so take this medication and let's wait and see if it worsens." Typically, while the patient goes home to wait, the

fibroids would grow bigger and may aggravate signs and symptoms, especially if she is on birth control pills.

2. Prayers and Holy Communion. For with God, all things are possible. He is our Healer. To me, fibroids have both medical and spiritual attachments, and therefore, they must be handled holistically. Matthew 9:20-22.

3. Having sex regularly. Some people revealed that their doctors told them to be having sex regularly to heal fibroids depending on the gravity of the symptoms of the fibroids.

4. Having a baby. Since fibroids can be a major cause affecting women's fertility and implantation, some doctors may advise their patients to start trying for a baby a few weeks or months after a fibroid surgery (Myomectomy).

5. Hormone Therapy, Birth Control Pills, Ibruprofen, Tranexamic Acid, Vitamins, Tot'he'ma- Blood Tonic and more.

6. Physical exercises and resorting to a positive lifestyle because your lifestyle affects the growth of fibroids.

7. Conventional medicines, herbal medicines, healthy diets, healthy living, seeds and nuts, eating foods

that are rich in fibre, and indulging in mild regular exercises every day.

8. Surround yourself with people that will care and support you. (Apply Self-Care and wellness practices)

9. Manage stress - There are possibilities that stress, anxiety and depression can trigger the growth of fibroids and cause them to grow larger, therefore, women suffering from fibroids must consciously learn how to lower and manage stress.

10. Menopause – After menopause, the estrogen level begins to drop, causing menstrual period to stop. With this, the fibroids will start to shrink naturally.

SIX DIAGNOSTIC SCANS OR TESTS FOR WOMEN SUFFERING FROM FIBROIDS

1. Pelvic Scan/Magnetic Resonance Imaging (MRI)/ Transvaginal scan: To know the size of the uterus, ovarian size, uterine lesion size and location, and the endometrial thickness in order to know the size and location of the fibroids.

2. Prolactin Test: This test is to diagnose and help find the cause of the abnormalities, irregularities or infertility.

3. Estrogen Test: This type of test helps to measure the level of estrogens which play a very important role in a female's menstruation, pregnancy, puberty and menopause.

4. Progesterone Test: This test helps to measure the level of progesterone. A hormone that is also important in the female reproductive system.

5. Luteinizing Hormone (LH) Test: This test helps to measure the amount of luteinizing hormone.

6. Blood count / Blood level Test: This test helps to measure the woman's red blood cells or the amount of blood level in her system. This test is very important, especially for women experiencing prolonged or heavy bleeding.

COME TO THE DOCTOR FULLY PREPARED

Most often, women walk into the doctor's office with little or no knowledge about the fibroid condition, just like I was. The Bible says, "My people are destroyed for lack of knowledge" Hosea 4:6. Before seeing your doctor or gynaecologist, ensure that you have prepared yourself enough to answer his or her diagnostic questions, and also, ask your own informative questions. I will advise you to take records of signs or symptoms that you have been experiencing, it will help in your treatments.

SEVEN POSSIBLE QUESTIONS YOUR DOCTOR MAY ASK YOU ON YOUR FIRST APPOINTMENT.

1 When was your last period?

2. How long do you have your period /what is the colour of your period?

3. Are your periods heavy or longer?

4. Do you feel pain when having intercourse?

5. How long have you been experiencing the heavy bleeding?

6. Have you been on any medication or seen any doctor about it?

7. Is there any family member with a fibroid history?

TEN QUESTIONS TO ASK YOUR DOCTOR ABOUT FIBROIDS AND THEIR TREATMENTS

1. What are fibroids /what type of tests or scans do I need to do?

2. If the tests and scans have been conducted, ask your doctor; what are the sizes and locations of the fibroids?

3. Do I need treatment right now or later?

4. What are the best options or treatments for me?

5. Are there options apart from surgery?

6. What are the risks involved in surgery?

7. What are the chances that the fibroids will not return after the surgery/ treatments?

8. What should I expect after the surgery/ treatments?

9. If I want to get pregnant, is it possible for me to get pregnant after the surgery or treatments?

10. How can I prevent the fibroids from returning?

CHAPTER 8

SELF-CARE & WELLNESS PRACTICES TO MANAGE FIBROIDS

I thank God for all the doctors, nurses and medical personnel who are doing their best in taking care of women suffering from fibroids, may God continue to bless them.

The Bible says, "Then you will know the truth, and the truth will set you free." John 8:32. One single truth that will help women suffering from fibroids to be free is to know about self-care and practice it.

What is self-care?

Self-care is a DELIBERATE or INTENTIONAL effort to focus on oneself without feeling guilty. It is the act of caring for one's health spiritually, physically and emotionally (One's personal well-being) in order for one to be able to take care of others. As the Bible says, "Love your neighbour as yourself."

Self-care practices are the golden rule for a happy environment and lifestyle. When an individual is burned-out, it means that the individual lacks and needs self-care practices. Don't ignore the red flags of self-care practices.

Women living with symptomatic fibroids often feel burnt out and unhappy because of the pains and discomforts that we experience regularly, and so, the need to practice self-care.

After several years of battling with that monster called fibroid, I became very desperate to find ways to take charge of my life and my health rather than just leaving my healthcare in the hands of doctors. Through research, I discovered self-care practices and I started implementing them. I made a promise to myself to start taking good care of my health, and this has helped me in the fibroid journey. By the grace of God, today, I am now happy because I am able to manage my health, and I can boldly say that fibroids can be treated and managed holistically through self-care practices, a healthy lifestyle, medically and herbal remedies.

Remember that treating and managing fibroids depends on the location and size of the fibroids. If you are experiencing signs and symptoms of fibroids, do not wait till they get worse, take charge of your health and seek medical assistance because early detection will save your life and womb.

Take charge of your health

You are completely responsible for your health and life, so refuse to make excuses or blame others and endeavour to make progress towards your health goals. As the saying goes "Health is Wealth".

If you fail to set health goals, you will be eating and drinking just anything that comes your way. Learn to set healthy boundaries for the sake of your well-being. "You are what you eat".

Most people are worried about falling sick, but they are not doing anything to protect their health, and this narrative must change. If you want to live a healthy life, you must spend time and effort to take charge of your health.

Brain Tracy, a management consultant once said, "One of the greatest benefits of setting a goal is that it enables you to control the direction of your life."

I know it is not easy to make the necessary change in your life, but I want you to know that it is possible and you can do it. Remember that "If you don't joyfully pay attention to your wellness today, you will painfully pay attention to your sickness tomorrow". It will not be our portion in Jesus' name. Amen!

If you neglect taking care of your health today, remember that when you get sick and die, life still goes on without you. "Life is a jungle," so fight to live a healthy life.

Keep in mind that the battle against fibroids can be very rough and tough, therefore, I encourage every woman battling with fibroids to be strong and of good courage. Also, be nice to yourself, buy yourself gifts, and let your self-talk be of only positive words. Sometimes you may feel like giving up, not wanting to take your medications and wellness practices, but do not stop, keep pressing on and remember that you can defeat fibroids and start living a happy life again. Your health is your treasure, so fight for it and be there for yourself. You need yourself; your family and society need you too. Don't see fibroid as a death sentence, but rather, perceive it as a health condition that can be managed and defeated. Encourage yourself as often as you can.

Bible says, *"David was greatly distressed because the men were talking of stoning him; each one was bitter in spirit because of his sons and daughters. But David found strength in the Lord his God." 1 Samuel 30:6.*

My dear, let me tell you something, I have cried several times without number during my battle with that monster called fibroid, but I have learned to encourage myself in the Lord, so I charge you not to drop your weapon of faith, your medications and self-care practices in the fight against fibroids, and by God's grace, you will win this battle. Say a big Amennnnnnnnnnnnnnnnnnnnn!

If you still believe in God for the fruit of the womb, keep on believing, for your miracle baby is on the way. Happy yourself; whether with a child or not, you deserve to be happy, don't you? Come on my sister, there is more to life. Turn your pain into passion and be a blessing to your generation. Don't let society stigmatize and throw you into darkness because you don't have a child. They are not God, okay? Most of them don't understand the fact that fibroids can affect women's fertility which is beyond our control. I send you hugs, okay? Be strong in the Lord, keep on praying and seek medical advice always.

Pay attention to these ten dimensions of wellness by the World Health Organization (WHO)

Ten Dimensions of Wellness.

These ten wellness dimensions are interrelated, so if you neglect one, it will affect the others.

1. "Physical dimensions
2. Nutritional dimensions
3. Medical dimensions
4. Social dimensions
5. Occupational dimensions
6. Behavioral dimensions
7. Emotional/psychological dimensions
8. Environmental dimensions
9. Financial dimensions
10. Spiritual dimensions'

Credit to Health Organization (WHO)

12 Things That I Did When I Took Charge Of My Health

Below are the other means that I deployed in managing and treating fibroids, though they are not scientifically proven. Always consult your doctors, and do not try to take the medications listed below because what works for me might not work for you.

1. I always consult my doctors for medical advice, and I constantly remind myself that nobody will lend me their body to live in, so I have to take good care of myself.

2. Detoxification of my body regularly.

3. I began to have a plan for my diet, "you are what you eat."

4. Castrol oil pack and hot water bottle.

5. Eating fruits and vegetables as often as I can.

6. Avoid red meat except otherwise.

7. Eat more fatty fish like mackerel, tuna and salmon.

8. Exercise as often as I can.

9. I started incorporating nuts and seeds into my diet as snacks.

10. Download the period tracking app.

11. Yoni (vaginal) steam with herbs.

12. Making my own juice and smoothies.

13. Drinking Apple cider vinegar and black strap molasses.

14. Drinking of "Prekese" /Tetraplewre, /Tetraptera tea

15. Drinking lots of water

16. Stress management

17. Sleeping well

Herbs / Leaves / Roots

1. Shepherd pursue

2. Dandelion/leaves

3. Raspberry

4. Yarrow

5. Aloe Vera

6. Maca root

7. Wild yam

8. Cinnamon leaves/ Powder

9. Vitex

10. Turmeric

11. Ginger

12. Garlic

13. Omega Fibroid Remover Herbal Solution

14. Beets

15. Tiger nuts

Medicinal Tea

1. Green tea

2. Fibroid tea

3. Tetrapleura Tetraptra (Prekese) tea

Other Home Remedies

1. Yoga
2. Massage of the womb/uterus
3. Acupuncture

Seed/nuts

1. Pumpkin seed
2. Sunflower
3. Sesame
4. Flax seed
5. Black seed
6. Cashew nut
7. Ground nut
8. Honey (sweetener)

Essential oils & Pack

1. Black seed oil
2. Castrol oil
3. Hot water bottle – Applying the heat on my lower belly

Supplements and Vitamins

1 Birth Control Pills, Ibruprofen, Tranexamic Acid, Tot'he'ma Blood Tonic

2. PMS with B6 & other B-vitamins

3. Organic Ashwagandha

3. Omega 3 Fish Oil

4. Zinc

5. Vitamin D-3 & K-2

6. Vitamin E

CHAPTER 9

30 PRAYER POINTS FOR FEMININE WELLNESS AGAINST FIBROIDS

What is Feminine Wellness? Is the holistic wellness of the most sacred part of the woman's body, which is the understanding of the wellness of the vaginal and the uterus/womb.

"Dear friend, I pray that you may enjoy good health and that all may go well with you, even as your soul is getting along well." (3 John 2)

Start by asking God for His forgiveness, and sing praises and worship songs, then say these prayer points with faith:

1. In the name of Jesus, I overcome every fibroid in my body.

2. Let the blood of Jesus flush out fibroids and abdominal sickness from my body.

3. In the name of Jesus, let every evil plantation of fibroid cast in my body be uprooted and die.

4. I soak my vagina, my womb in the blood of Jesus.

5. Holy Ghost, as I clap my hands, let every demonic altar fighting my wellness be broken in Jesus' name.

6. Oh Lord my God, send your healing hand to touch my body right now from any reproductive health problem like fibroids, endometriosis, ovarian cysts, vaginal cancer, irregular periods, polycystic ovary syndrome(PCOS), sexually transmitted diseases (STDs), vesico vaginal fistula (VVF) etc. They should all die by the fire of the holy ghost.

7. In the name of Jesus, I arrest every power fighting my womb.

8. Every arrow of sickness and death, be broken right now.

9. I claim divine healing and freedom from every sickness in Jesus' name.

10. In the name of Jesus, I divorce myself and my family from every familiar spirit.

11. I break the hold of all demonic powers over my life in the name of Jesus.

12. You spirit of bleeding, leave my body now in Jesus' name.

13. O Lord, my Healer and Helper, let your presence circulate every part of my reproductive system right now.

14. In the name of Jesus, let every dead organ in my reproductive system receive life right now.

15. By the power in the name of Jesus, I set myself free from evil patterns operating in my family.

16. O Lord Jesus, stretch out your mighty hand into my life and let it receive the fruits of the womb right now.

17. My father, let me not be put to shame in Jesus' name.

18. Lord, let every food that I eat and water that I drink be a blessing and heal my body in Jesus' name.

19. Let every medication that I take heal me from fibroids.

20. By the blood of Jesus, let the doctor's hands be touched anytime I visit the hospital. I cover all

medical officers that will attend to me in the hospital with the blood of Jesus.

21. I am fertile in Jesus' name.

22. I refuse to wear any demonic garments of sorrow, hormonal imbalances and depression in Jesus' name.

23. O Lord, liberate me from any unhidden family curse and sickness.

24. I reject any anti-marriage and anti-healing power over my life.

25. In the name of Jesus, let family ones be filled with God's power and healing.

26. I bind, uproot and paralyse any assigned demons over my life.

27. I command my reproductive system to reject any evil plantation of sickness.

28. I drink the blood of Jesus.

29. I thank you Lord for your healing power over my life and family. Let your power overshadow my family and me.

30. Lord, I give you glory and thank you for my victory over my sickness because you live. I am an overcomer. End with songs of praise.

CHAPTER 10

---

31 DAYS WELLNESS AFFIRMATION SCRIPTURES TO COMFORT FIBROIDS PATIENTS

Day 1

"Fear not; for I am with you: be not dismayed; for I am your God: I will strengthen you, I will help you, I will uphold you with my righteous right hand." (Isaiah 41:10)

Day 2

"So we do not lose heart, though our outer self is wasting away, our inner self is being renewed day by day. For this light momentary affliction is preparing for us an eternal weight of glory." (2 Corinthians 4: 16-18)

Day 3

"Even though I walk through the valley of the shadow of death, I will fear no evil, for you are with me; your rod and staff they comfort me." (Psalm 23:4)

Day 4

"Cast your burden on the Lord, and he will sustain you; He will never permit the righteous to be rumoured." (Psalm 55:22)

Day 5

"Come to me, all who labour and are heavy laden and I will give you rest. Take my yoke upon you, and learn from me, for I am gentle and lowly in heart and you will find rest." (Matthew 11:28-29)

Day 6

"And he said unto me, my grace is sufficient for these; for my strength is made perfect in weakness. Most gladly in my infirmities, which the power of Christ may rest upon me." (2 Corinthians 12:9)

Day 7

"Be strong and courageous, do not fear or be in dread of them, for it is the Lord your God who goes with you.

He will not leave you nor forsake you." (Deuteronomy 31:6)

Day 8

"For I know the plans I have for you declares the Lord, plans to prosper you and met to harm you, plans to give you hope and future." (Jeremiah 29:11)

Day 9

"When you pass through the water, I will be with you; and when you pass through the rivers, they will not sweep you over, when you walk through the fire you will not be burned, the flames will not set you ablaze." (Isaiah 43:2)

Day 10

"Do not be afraid, for I am with you…" (Isaiah 43:5)

Day 11

"The Lord is close to the brokenhearted…" (Psalm 34:18)

Day 12

"In you, Lord my God I put my trust. I trust in you don't let me be put to shame, let not my enemies trample over me." (Psalm 25:1-2)

Day 13

"Ask and it will be given to you, seek and you will

find, knock and the door will be opened to you, for everyone who asks receives, the one who seeks finds, and to the one who knocks the door will be opened." (Matthew 7:7-8)

Day 14

"And I will do whatever you ask in my name so that the Father may be glorified in the Son." (John 14:13)

Day 15

"Peace I leave with you; my peace I give you; I do not give to you as the world gives. Do not let your heart be troubled and do not be afraid." (John 14:27)

Day 16

"Everyone who calls on the name of the Lord will be saved." (Romans 10:13)

Day 17

"However as it is written; what no eye has seen, what no ear has heard, and what no human mind has conceived; the things God has prepared for those who love him." (1 Corinthians 2:9)

Day 18

"My presence will go with you, and I will give you rest." (Exodus 33:14)

Day 19

"When the righteous cry for help, the Lord hears and rescues them from all their troubles." (Psalms 34:17)

Day 20

"I sought the Lord, and He answered me and delivered me from all my fears." (Psalm 34:4)

Day 21

"Surely God is my Salvation; I will trust and not be afraid. The Lord is my strength and my song he has become my salvation." (Isaiah 12:2)

Day 22

"My grace is sufficient for you, for my power is made perfect in weakness." (2 Corinthians 12:9)

Day 23

"But the Lord is faithful, and He will strengthen and protect you from the evil ones." (2 Thessalonians 3:3)

Day 24

"He gives power to the weak and strength to the powerless." (Isaiah 40:29)

Day 25

"Bless the Lord, O my soul, and forget not all His benefits. Who forgives all your iniquities, who heals all your diseases…" (Psalm 103:2-5)

Day 26

"Many are the afflictions of the righteous, but the Lord delivers him out of them all." (Psalm 34:19)

Day 27

"Behold, I will bring it health and healing, I will heal them and reveal to them the abundance of peace and truth." (Jeremiah 33:6)

Day 28

"The Lord will strengthen him on his bed of illness. You will sustain him on his sickbed." (Psalm 41:3)

Day 29

"O Lord my God. I cried out to you, and you healed me." (Psalm 30:2)

Day 30

"He heals the brokenhearted and binds up their wounds." (Psalm 147:3)

Day 31

"He was pierced for our transgression and by His stripes, we are healed." (Isaiah 53:5)

Aunty Fanny - May, 2015

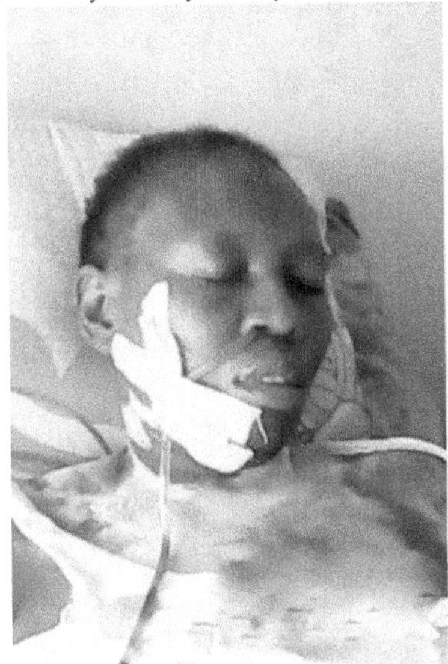 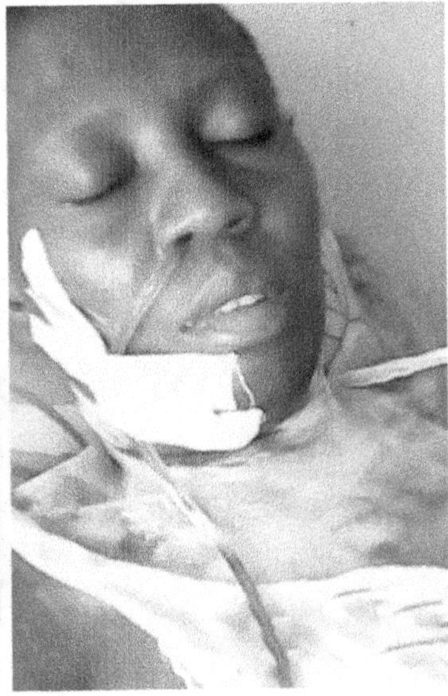

Aunty Fanny - Dec. 2022

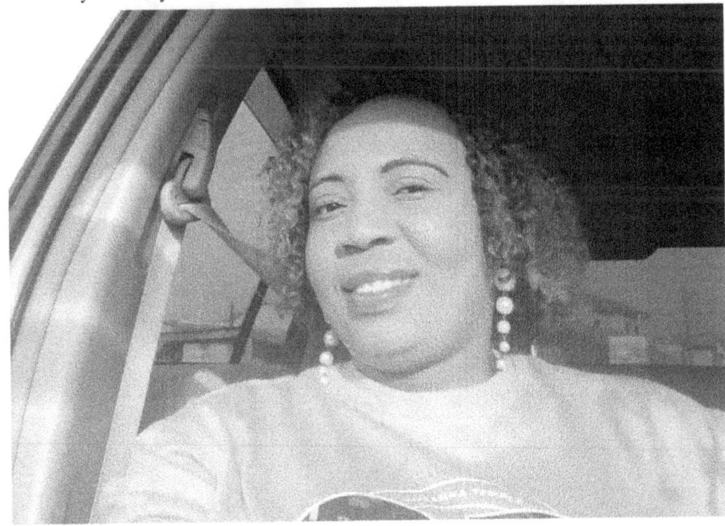

9 798860 502635